INSOMNIAC

Defeating Insomnia with
Tried-and-True Methods

Jennifer Schwarz

Disclaimer

Please note the information contained within this document is for educational purposes only. Every attempt has been made to provide accurate, up-to-date, reliable, and complete information. No warranties of any kind are expressed or implied. Readers acknowledge that the author is not engaging in the rendering of legal, financial, medical, or professional advice.

By reading this document, the reader agrees that under no circumstances are we responsible for any direct or indirect losses incurred as a result of misuse of information contained within this document, including, but not limited to, errors, omissions, or inaccuracies.

Table Of Contents

Introduction

Welcome to INSOMNIAC: The Ultimate Sleep Therapy book. This book includes tried-and-true methods for dealing with insomnia in all its facets, from its causes to its treatment. You may conquer the insomnia process with all the knowledge in this book.

All of the sleepless nights and all of the perpetually worn-out days will be forgotten. After reading this book, you will understand the causes of insomnia and how to treat it. Once again, I appreciate your support and wish you much success with this book.

Chapter 1

The Science of Insomnia

Have you ever experienced sleeplessness? Do you struggle to go to sleep and remain asleep at night, in other words? What, then, is the cause?

Insomnia often results from a combination of factors, including inadequate sleep, hunger, psychological stress, etc. Regardless of the cause, millions of people battle the demon known as insomnia. You are prevented from obtaining adequate sleep, your vitality is depleted, and your productivity the next day is ruined, not to mention the harm it does to your physical and psychological well-being.

What is Insomnia

By definition, insomnia is the inability to go to sleep and remain asleep. It describes the many kinds of restlessness a person has during their sleep cycle.

When a person feels dissatisfied with the quantity of sleep he or she has been obtaining, it is a sign of insomnia.

People who suffer from insomnia will have low energy levels, weariness at various times during the day, struggle to focus on activities, suffer from unpleasant mood swings, and perform poorly at work. These symptoms might occur in insomniacs after a night of unremitting vigilance.

The human body needs sleep to regenerate both the intellect and the body. The outcome of any of them getting too little sleep is exhaustion and various mental ailments. Many struggle to fall or remain asleep despite being tired for various reasons.

The Two Types of Insomnia

1. Acute Slumber

The two basic forms of insomnia are as follows. The first sort of insomnia is the kind that only lasts a few sleepless nights. You can often fall asleep and remain asleep with ease. Many insomniacs may not believe they have the condition, yet they may be experiencing acute insomnia.

What precisely is acute insomnia? This particular kind of insomnia results from the extreme amounts of stress that insomniacs are going through at the time. Due to the current conditions in their lives, individuals will experience a brief time during which they cannot fall asleep. This kind of sleeplessness does not last very long. Instead, it only occurs under certain conditions and at a specific time.

For example, insomniacs may have severe insomnia after facing their boss's fury, receiving a poor mark on a test, being rejected by their sweetheart, or simply because they are having a "Bad Day." These circumstances may lead to one or two nights when a person cannot sleep. This kind of insomnia is probably common and usually goes away by itself.

2. Chronic Sleepiness

Chronic insomnia is the name for the second form of insomnia. It is a chronic form of insomnia that lasts at least three months and affects at least three evenings each week. This usually happens when your environment—physically or mentally—is about to shift substantially. Moving to a new house, losing a loved one, starting a new job, dealing with difficulties in school, or struggling to adjust to harsher weather are just a few examples. Maybe chronic insomniacs struggle to sleep because they have an unhealthy sleeping pattern or lack a regular sleep schedule.

It's prevalent in today's environment; short sleep

durations have messed with the sleep cycle. Even worse, the majority of them sleep at strange hours. They don't have the routine of going to bed and getting up early every day.

Consequently, the mind would get used to staying late and not knowing when to turn off. Because of this, sleeplessness has spread across modern civilization. The body cannot operate with just a few hours of sleep in one night, and individuals often think that taking naps later in the day can compensate for their lack of sleep. While initially, this could appear feasible and helpful, this sleep pattern is not long-term maintainable.

The mind and body will eventually give out, and you won't feel fully recovered until you get enough sleep. The best remedy is following a regular sleep pattern and good sleep hygiene. If not, you must get prescription medicine from a doctor. Usually, it will be connected to another physical or psychological problem. Therefore, stress may be the cause of your persistent sleeplessness. If you have chronic insomnia, even an ordinary setting can feel stressful. Any input from the immediate surroundings will irritate a restless mind and body.

The Causes of Insomnia

The reasons for all forms of insomnia are the same. The distinction is in how strongly an individual feels for a certain period. In addition, undiagnosed medical disorders might also contribute to sleeplessness. Fortunately, most types of insomnia are curable.

These illnesses, which may be either severe or moderate, can cause insomnia at various times during a person's life. Nasal and sinus allergies, lower back discomfort, generalized chronic pain, gastrointestinal issues, arthritis, asthma, and other neurological issues are some of these symptoms.

The patient's mind will remain awake for longer due to the stress on their body. For instance, those with a cold may discover they wake up often or spend most of the night awake. A person may significantly lose sleep and rest due to both circumstances. They could attempt to unwind while sick with a cold, but sleeplessness will win.

The inability to get into a comfortable sleeping posture due to physical discomfort may also contribute to insomnia. Have you ever had trouble falling asleep because you couldn't find a comfortable position?

This is a regular scenario whenever you suffer physical discomfort. The key to falling and staying asleep quickly is to arrange your body comfortably in bed. It will also promote healing and provide a better night's sleep. Otherwise, if you can't get into your optimum position, you'll constantly struggle to fall asleep and may even decide to take unneeded medicine. We can turn to the remedy now that we know all these distinct causes. But it's as crucial to research all the elements.

Induce slumber. But did you realize that insomnia

also has risk factors? You simply have a larger likelihood of experiencing insomnia at some time in your life if you discover that any of these factors apply to you. If not, be mindful of your well-being and sleeping patterns to prevent insomnia for the rest of your life.

The Insomnia Risk Factors

The risk factors for insomnia include:
- Being a woman, pregnant, or going through menopause.
- Individuals over 40.
- Experiencing increased stress or sadness.
- Working nights.
- Traveling long distances with a time shift.
- Having a history of the condition in your family.

Each of these causes brings us one step closer to sleeplessness. However, are you aware that most of these risk factors are a consequence of your decisions? People often believe they have little to no control over their lives, yet this is untrue.

When traveling across several time zones, they could take a longer vacation but choose not to. They could have chosen to work during the day, but they chose to endure the hardships of a nighttime job and adjust to a new way of life.

Although managing the sleeplessness risk factors might be challenging, ultimately, your decisions will determine how you go. You could have difficult periods in life sometimes. Relationship issues, family issues, or employment issues may all be contributors. Additionally, you could be experiencing difficulties juggling your personal and work lives due to financial or other issues. Until most of the stress or despair has subsided, these will harass and keep you up at night. It can take longer in certain circumstances. Other times, individuals can rapidly overcome difficulties and discover answers. In any case, the solution to emotions-caused sleeplessness has the appropriate mentality.

You may do many things to stop yourself from experiencing sleepless and restless nights since insomnia has many causes and risk factors. Most of the time, determining the reasons is simple; the real issue is doing so while still getting a decent night's sleep. Life can be challenging, and occasionally it may bring someone to the point where he doubts his ability to rise again.

Being courageous is the first and most important step in combating insomnia. Do not fear potential consequences or effects that may or may not occur. Your life becomes more stressful due to fear, which is unhealthy. In reality, it will just make your sleeplessness worse. Prevention is always preferable to treatment. Keep your cool and adhere to the health advice to avoid experiencing insomnia.

Chapter 2

The Mind of an Insomniac

Researchers from all around the globe are collaborating to understand how an insomniac's brain functions. They are still examining the characteristics of each brainwave and the interactions between thoughts throughout the day and night.

How the Mind Functions

The mind can change to any brand-new circumstance at any time of the day. The mind continuously seeks novel strategies for surviving and thriving, whether you're attempting to get food, or a drink, exit a moving vehicle, pass through a door, or just find some rest. The cycle of acquiring adequate resources during the day and having enough energy for recovery and slumber during the night will continue.

Normal brainwave activity and enough cognitive

stability over the day enable individuals to normally shut off certain mental processes. Processes that happen during the night. The brain will start to slow down and commence sleep as darkness falls deeper. At night, you often become less focused and alert. This is the cause of why doing anything at night is more difficult.

According to studies, the mental processes normally alter during the day and might sometimes result in severe anxiety. When much stress occurs throughout the day, the brainwaves become irregular and won't calm down. As a result, the mind won't be able to sleep deeply at night. The brainwaves will instead experience a time of exceptionally rapid movement, which will result in more thoughts and need more energy in the evening. At night, a person will remember everything that happened throughout the day. The body will then use twice as much energy and resources to process the ideas, which results in exhaustion and poor energy the next day.

The Brainwaves And The Mind

Three studies demonstrate how the brain behaves at night concerning thoughts and how the brainwaves react to the stages of insomnia. It has been shown that a person's sleep is impacted by how their brain learns and processes memories. Your brain will process more ideas and memories at night as you gain more knowledge throughout the day.

Dreams are the result of one's ideas and experiences in reality. You dream more at night the more life experiences you have. The capacity for a greater range of dreams enables the mind to settle down and create hazy pictures to help you remember things. You often have dreams while you are fast asleep. You could even have nightmares sometimes. But it all comes down to this. Down to the kind of encounter you experienced and your repressed ideas.

Night vs. Day

So what goes on in insomniacs' brains? First, their brains have greater activity at night and have a harder time relaxing and quiet. Scientists have shown that the brain's neurons of insomniacs are more active at night in one of their investigations on the brainwaves during sleep deprivation.

People who suffer from insomnia often have many things running through their minds. They are in a continual state of information processing during the whole day without being able to stop it. They'll eventually get insomnia and deal with the effects of getting little sleep.

According to experts, insomnia shouldn't be considered just a condition of the night. It's more of a 24-hour brain disorder that keeps the brain working all day.

Memory processing and archiving are significantly influenced by sleep. Sleep deprivation will eventually affect your memory. You'll struggle to focus and recall information and even tiny details. On a brief exam, a group of students were used to test this notion. While one group slept through the previous night, the other did not. The outcomes? More rested students could better concentrate and remember their exam answers many hours later. Students who didn't get enough sleep had trouble with the exam, had below-average results, and had trouble remembering their answers an hour later.

The Myths

This experiment demonstrates how crucial rest is to one's ability to concentrate and retain information. Those who suffer from insomnia can't focus to the same degree as people who get adequate sleep. Unexpectedly, some individuals think they can maintain the same focus throughout the day, even if the brain is just as busy at night as during the day. This does not necessarily imply that it can perform at its best.

According to a study, insomniacs have greater

brain flexibility than others. But the study of what plasticity is and how it's yet unclear how it affects the states of sleeplessness. However, they understand that as a person ages, their brain's plasticity increases and eventually plays a role in various types of illness. Brain plasticity is the brain's capacity to adapt physically and functionally in response to external or internal factors.

Brain plasticity often allows us to take in new knowledge, gain new skills, and continue to develop over time.

Adulthood. However, sleeplessness harms your brain's neurons and promotes brain plasticity. This causes a loss of attention and poor memory recall in the near term and the long run. As a person ages, it becomes harder to maintain all the levels of attention and memory.

The Restless Mind's Brain

Another study looked at how worry and stress

impact sleep. The objective was to ascertain if someone who leads a stressful lifestyle has insomnia and how their brain functions at night. The effect is that regardless of whether a person has insomnia, their brain's cognitive performance remains the same. Concentrating and digesting information during the day is more difficult for insomniacs.

Most studies indicate that people with insomnia have restless nights. The next day, they'll struggle to focus and have trouble juggling their job, academics, and personal life.

In other words, the mind will not work at its finest the next day, and insomniacs cannot function at their best. In another section of the study, the recollection of insomniacs and those who get adequate sleep can function and work efficiently to do any assigned duties.

According to studies, insomniacs have trouble remembering most of their daily recollections.

They struggle to do their everyday responsibilities as a consequence. Even while they are doing basic things, their thoughts would wander. For instance, people who get sufficient sleep will go to the kitchen, make rapid decisions, and begin their day. Those who are experiencing insomnia, on the other hand, will go into the kitchen, end up opening more cupboards, browse through the same items, and end up unable to decide what they should have for breakfast!

And here is why: Because an insomniac's brainwaves are slower, he or she will move more slowly and lose basic information more rapidly. Additionally, as the day goes on and more duties are assigned to them, the prefrontal cortex will start to have fewer resources, which will cause the brainwaves to become unpredictable. The brain will try to continue functioning, but it won't have the energy to do so. Therefore, if you have insomnia, your brain will ultimately get exhausted.

The Grey Area

The third and last scientific investigation will look at the function of the grey matter in the brain. The fact that grey matter is located in the frontal lobe and regulates memory and executive function is the most crucial fact to understand about it.

Insomniacs' grey matter will significantly shrink if they don't sleep enough at night. They will gradually start to show signs of depression or trauma, whether they have insomnia or generally have difficulties sleeping. Stress is often the root cause of sleeplessness. A doctor's advice on the right medication for you is the best action for dealing with this problem.

Simply said, the mind needs enough sleep and rest to concentrate well. Your body will only go into overdrive if you have insomnia, preventing you from obtaining proper rest. Getting proper nourishment and sleep each night is the next critical point to remember. No matter how difficult it may be to strike a balance, it's critical to maintain a high level of focus each day to make the most of your time.

Chapter 3

Sleep-deprived - The Devil

The previous chapter examined the mind to comprehend the direct effects of insomnia on the brain. The mind will suffer greatly if this condition persists for any time. In addition to memory loss, insomnia causes fatigue, carelessness, and lack of attentiveness the next day. Rest is essential for a healthy mind and body the following day. Without sleep, the brain's intricate functions, like memory and reasoning, will deteriorate, making it impossible for insomniacs to function throughout the day. They will battle to maintain concentration all day as their thoughts constantly stray.

The 5 Things You Perform Each Morning

Here's a quick exercise: First, attempt to recall everything you did as soon as you awoke today. Think back on the first five actions you took. The alarm clock may be turned off, the phone might be checked, and you might get up, turn on the lights, and go to the restroom. You tend to carry out all your daily tasks perfectly, regardless of your typical schedule. Unbelievably, you carry out all of these tasks automatically and without much thinking, since they have become a part of your everyday routine.

However, you are not quite as concentrated as usual when you have insomnia. The mind will keep thinking as soon as possible.

As it typically would, but it lacks the resources and energy necessary to do so. In other words, you could struggle to finish each of the first five things you must do in the morning.

Knowing when you notice it takes longer than it ought to complete these duties is a simple method. If you didn't get enough sleep, the five tasks that should only take two minutes to accomplish might require more than ten. Even worse, you could overlook one or two tasks. It's possible that you won't remember to turn off the alarm or check your phone for new messages. When you have insomnia, many different things might occur, but this is merely the tip of the iceberg.

Your Professional Life Being Affected

Your energy level may noticeably decline after the first night of dealing with insomnia. You could find it more difficult to recall everything you learn during the day or that it's harder to arrange your day.

Your typical daily routine can start with getting out of bed, getting ready for work, or even shopping. Demand complete concentration to guarantee high levels of performance and effectiveness. Otherwise, your employer could give you the finger. No matter how worn out you may be, you will only get pity for a few days. You are only permitted a certain number of sick days each year. Don't allow sleeplessness to ruin your relationships with family, friends, and coworkers.

Take control and permanently get rid of it.

You are required to do the responsibilities for your employment by a certain date. You have to be at the top of your game practically every day, whether in charge of writing, researching, or packing boxes. You must always provide your best effort to get your well-earned salary at the end of the month. Any sleep loss throughout the night might lead to poor performance the following day.

Do You Feel Sleep Deficient?

Although each person has a different sleep cycle, doctors advise getting 6 to 8 hours daily. The precise figure varies depending on the person. Some of us need more sleep than others. But ultimately, sacrificing a few hours of sleep is always preferable to losing a whole night. For instance, rather than purchasing, you only get six hours of sleep instead of eight. Even if those two hours of sleep can seem essential, they won't affect your life as negatively as insomnia. Losing two hours of sleep could make you less productive, but you'll probably be able to persevere and finish all your duties by the end of the day. On the other side, not getting enough sleep might cause your brain to shut down. They will have a difficult day doing basic activities.

For instance, you have no trouble reading the text of an agenda when your boss places it on your desk. Understanding what each item on the list signifies is challenging for folks who suffer from insomnia. What seems to be a simple task for those suffering from insomnia could be difficult.

Lack of sleep often causes you to lose concentration and direction for the day. Instead of considering the greatest method to go through the day, you continually seek the quickest route. Because you sometimes still manage to do tasks on time, it could first appear reasonable. In actuality, however, your reputation at work will suffer in the long term due to your subpar job. Additionally, insomniacs are noted for having a short fuse and difficulty getting along with their coworkers.

People will soon become aware of your inefficiencies. Your manager will see that you are working more slowly, not paying as close attention, and not in the proper frame of mind to do the task. It may make your supervisor dislike you, and you risk losing your job. Although it may now seem implausible, you should know that the likelihood is quite high. A troubling aspect of life, insomnia may interfere with a person's personal and professional relationships.

Your Personal Life Being Damaged

Consider everything that is significant to you and that you hold dear to your heart as you consider your personal life. You could consider your wife, spouse, kids, pets, or other factors. Some individuals may even consider their yard or the renovation job they have been working on.

There is no correct or incorrect response to this. It's your life; achieving success depends on keeping a healthy balance. Most individuals go about their regular activities without giving them much attention. Examples of this are easy actions like putting the kids' breakfast together, getting in the vehicle, or heading out to dinner.

Normal people wouldn't consider their challenging jobs, but insomniacs could disagree. When a person's personal life deviates from equilibrium, it causes stressful situations, and they start to wonder whether there is a method to return to a steady state.

No matter where the tension is coming from—not having the groceries in time or getting up late—even a little bit of stress may build up to become unmanageable. Significant amounts of tension and tiredness are brought on by insomnia.

They won't have any particular ideas; instead, their minds will roam and think meaningless, random things. The same holds for their professional lives. If you have insomnia and need to get your kids ready for school, you can forget to pack their lunches, straighten their clothing, etc.

Remember that "Self-Love is NOT Selfish," and put yourself first. When you consistently put yourself last, your life will spiral downhill, and you won't be able to achieve your ultimate goal.

Now is the moment to dispel a major myth in our culture: the idea that putting oneself first is conceited, bad, and selfish. They overlooked that if you spend your time attending to the needs of others without pursuing your own goals, you will feel unhappy and doomed. If you go this route, you'll lose your zeal, inspiration, passion, and productivity. Therefore, stop trying to please others and put yourself first. You won't be able to stop yourself from doing more and giving more in return until you do this.

You may need to do maintenance tasks around

your property, such as mowing the grass and looking for pests. You must always remember the procedures to properly carry out each activity. When you have insomnia, you won't be able to recall things very well and will find it more difficult to complete tasks.

Your interpersonal relationships are an important aspect of your personal life as well. Being in a relationship is a work in and of itself, whether with your spouse, boyfriend, girlfriend, or any other kind of partner. Your relationship may suffer if you cannot focus completely on your lover because you aren't getting enough sleep. This condition will result from arguments, discontent, anger, loneliness, and melancholy in a relationship. All of these feelings have the potential to get so out of control that a significant confrontation may be required.

Managing Insomnia

When you have no more energy, dealing with sleeplessness is difficult. You'll always feel worn out and less interested in what is happening in the world. Your ideas will sometimes become illogical when your mind wanders. Life is difficult enough as it is. Imagine now that you must also cope that you are not getting any rest and that life has presented you with various challenges. What would you think? Overwhelmed? Stressed?

You may waste time at work. You risk upsetting your kids by forgetting to prepare family dinners. You risk beginning to overlook all the little details. Typically carried out for your intimate partnership. Insomnia may cause many aspects of your life to fail. Keeping this in mind, It's time to prevent sleep loss and ensure you always receive the best possible sleep.

Chapter 4
The Cure: Natural and Artificial Treatments

Sleep is crucial for good health. Our bodies need sleep to recover and reenergize after the day's events. Insomnia cures are helpful since, regrettably, many individuals either have trouble falling asleep or don't get enough sleep.

When it comes to insomnia remedies, there are two groups.

1. Artificial Fix

The Artificial Remedy comes first. Both the drugstore and the clinic carry this kind of treatment or medication. They are often given to treat illnesses at their root. Although artificial remedies can cost a fortune, they frequently provide quick benefits. Most modern medications are poisonous and include dangerous substances that should not be ingested over an extended period.

2. Natural Cure

The second kind of cure is referred to as a natural remedy. People have used natural medicine for millennia. This treatment uses the body's innate ability to repair itself to combat insomnia. Although they are often less costly, what sets them apart is the fact that they are less hazardous than Artificial Remedies.

Regardless of the cure you choose, the objective is to make it easier for you to get and remain asleep. These treatments are intended to help you sleep better at night. Unless otherwise specified, taking these medications immediately before bed is preferable since most of them will make you drowsy. Additionally, seeing a doctor before using any of the following medications is critical.

1. Eszopiclone, sometimes referred to as Lunesta belongs to a class of medications that may put you

to sleep fast and comfortably. According to statistics, Lunesta may help most individuals fall asleep for an average of 7 to 8 hours. It's a potent class of medications, so avoid using it unless you can get a full night's sleep to avoid drowsiness. The FDA prohibits medication dosages of more than 1 mg. Any more might increase the likelihood of feeling sleepy the next day.

2. Ramelteon: This class of medications works differently; it doesn't give consumers unpleasant side effects like grogginess or sleepiness. The CNS (Central Nervous System) is the target of common medicines used to induce sleep, suppressing its functioning and putting the user to sleep. On the other hand, Ramelteon especially targets the sleep-wake cycle. This medication is recommended for those who have trouble falling asleep. Ramelteon may be used for a long time since it has no negative effects. The medicine hasn't previously been associated with misuse or dependency.

3. Sonata and Zaleplon are similar terms. Most medications take a long time to activate in the human body. One of them is not a sonata. Sonata has the shortest duration of activity in the body out of all the most recent sleeping medicines. In other words, the morning after taking this medication, there are minimal to no negative effects. For instance, taking a Sonata tablet may assist someone who has trouble getting asleep and keep them from feeling groggy the following day.

4. Also known as Silenor, doxepin. Those who have trouble remaining asleep are especially given this class of medications. You might argue that this is a man-made treatment for "light-sleepers" who often wake up throughout the night due to a little bit of light.

It is a stimulus. It works by blocking the histamine receptors, which help you stay asleep after falling asleep. Do not use Silenor unless you can sleep for 7-8 hours at night since this medication demands you to remain asleep for a certain period. Your age, health, and reaction to therapy all factor into the dose.

5. Benzodiazepines: Both short-term and long-term insomnia may be treated with benzodiazepines. Given how long it remains in the system, it has an ongoing impact on the body. Therefore, this medication may help folks who have experienced insomnia for a long time get well.

It is often used to treat sleepwalking and protracted nightmares. The uncompromising nature of this drug's impact may cause you to feel sleepy and worn out the following day. Another negative effect of this prescription is the potential for drug dependency, which might mean that you eventually need to rely on it to help you fall and remain asleep.

Triazolam (Halcion), Alprazolam (Xanax), Temazepam (Restoril), among other sleeping medicines, include benzodiazepines.

Before using any sleeping medications, getting a medical checkup is essential. For a full evaluation, see a doctor. Always

Before choosing which tablets to take, speak with your doctor about any possible side effects of the drugs you want to take. Each medication has potential adverse effects that vary. A headache, a strong allergic response, and protracted sleepiness are just a few of the negative effects.

However, some people would rather turn to natural treatments. You don't need to rely on substances that have dangerous side effects, particularly when you first wake up. Use natural solutions to restore your sleep cycle and eliminate insomnia instead.

1. Go Camping

It's time to pack up the tent and go camping if watching TV or playing with your phone keeps you up late at night. Avoid using electronics and sometimes indulge in a digital detox. Be attentive to your surroundings and yourself, and create a distraction-free environment. Use this time to practice yoga, write, journal, reflect, or breathe. According to multiple studies, campers who avoid technology and engage in relaxing routines like meditation or music listening go to bed around two hours earlier than normal. One other crucial thing to keep in mind is that digital gadgets.

Contribute to sleeplessness. It has been discovered that artificial light sources may harm circadian rhythms.

Instead of sleeping in your vehicle or camper, try sleeping outside. You'll become grounded and at one with nature in this manner. No matter what you do when camping, the main objective is to unwind, escape people's expectations and distractions, avoid artificial light, and connect with nature. When the sun goes down, take a bath in the natural sunlight. You'll quickly readjust your sleep patterns.

2. Music Therapy

Since ancient times, people have employed music to treat sleeplessness. It is a therapeutic technique that may aid in reducing anxiety, which can affect the quality of your sleep. This method's main benefit is its simple use and has no negative side effects.

Music treatments come in various forms and vary in the kinds of neurological stimulation they elicit. For instance, although rock music may be uncomfortable, classical music may be a strong instrument for comfort and relaxation. Choose soothing music with natural sounds like the ocean, birds, waterfalls, etc.

According to many studies, those who listen to relaxing music before bed sleep better than those who don't. Consequently, this may be the answer if you have difficulties falling asleep.

3. Switch off for better sleep

There is no on/off switch for sleep. Your body needs time to relax and get ready for sleep. It might be challenging for insomniacs to turn off their brains at night. Try turning off the lights for better sleep. This method helps to calm things down so that your body will recognize that it is time to rest. It's important to relax and let our minds wander before bed.

For instance, taking a warm before bed can cause your body's temperature to decrease, which will signal your body to begin preparing for sleep. You may raise your body's temperature by taking a warm shower.

Reduce the pace of respiration, digestion, and heartbeat to slow down metabolic processes. Your body will realize that it is time to unwind and calm down. Your body will get conditioned to believe that listening to music at night means it is time to go to bed if you make it a practice to do so.

It all comes down to training and habits. Spend at least 30 minutes relaxing before going to bed by practising deep breathing or other relaxation techniques. Your brain is supposed to get a signal during this power-down hour that it is time to wind down, relax, and go to bed.

4. Sleep in a cool place

Compared to their healthy counterparts, those who have trouble going to sleep often have a greater core body temperature just before falling asleep. This group of insomniacs must thus wait for at least two to four hours before their body temperatures drop and sleep begins.

According to studies, a room's ideal temperature for sleep is between 16 and 20 degrees Celsius. Your brain likes it cool while you're attempting to fall asleep.

Additionally, sleeping in a cool bedroom slows the ageing process. It facilitates the release of melatonin, a powerful antioxidant that fights inflammation, boosts the immune system, and guards against cancer and cognitive decline. Melatonin is one of the body's anti-ageing hormones.

A proverb states that those who get up and sleep early live longer. It makes great sense since sleeping in a cool bedroom decreases oxidative stress and neurodegeneration. I could go on and on about how sleeping in a cool atmosphere has anti-ageing advantages. But getting enough sleep is essential for increasing the body's production of anti-ageing chemicals.

And the first step in doing that is to make the bedroom a comfortable temperature for sleeping. A lack of sleep has many negative repercussions on your physical and emotional well-being. In the end, it can endanger your life.

Your sleeping patterns, and you may start by setting up a comfortable sleeping space.

5. Break A Sweat

Early workouts. Exercise enhances general health and sleep. However, research published in the journal Sleep demonstrates that the volume and timing of exercise matter. According to research, women who work out at a moderate level for at least 30 minutes every morning, seven days a week, have fewer problems falling or staying asleep.

A later time today. Our biological rhythms seem to be favorably impacted by morning exercise, which enhances our sleep quality.

Body temperature may be one of the causes of this interaction between activity and sleep. Exercise causes an increase in body temperature, which takes up to 6 hours to return to normal. It's because greater sleep is associated with lower body temperatures. Therefore, allowing your body to calm down before bed is crucial.

Our ability to recover and maintain our health depends on sleep. Take it seriously, and if you're having trouble controlling your sleep, consider seeing a functional medicine specialist. All of these need dedication and self-control. You'll finally benefit from peaceful, restorative sleep after you reset your biological clock and return to the typical sleep schedule.

Chapter 5

Insomniac Lifestyle Modification

The preceding chapter covered the two main kinds of insomnia treatments. These extrinsic variables, however, could not address the underlying cause of sleeplessness. Yes, you could feel better after using such solutions, but insomnia won't be cured until the cause of the issue is addressed. Otherwise, there is a strong likelihood that sleeplessness will return.

Then what causes insomnia? For many people, having a bad lifestyle and poor sleeping habits is the main cause of insomnia. Simple lifestyle adjustments may significantly improve the quality of your sleep.

Although stress isn't the only factor in sleeplessness, it is obvious that chronically stressed individuals are more prone to insomnia. In a stressful situation,

Regarding insomnia, reducing or eliminating stress will make sleep easier. As noted in the book's first chapter, stress impacts how well a person sleeps, which might mess with their sleep cycle. Therefore, remaining awake throughout the day and falling asleep at night will be challenging.

To maintain a good balance in your life, it is crucial to manage every aspect of it as well as you can. The amount of sleep you receive each night must be adequate; you must ensure. Your physical health is greatly influenced by sleep. Short-term sleep deprivation may worsen your mood and irritability. Serious long-term complications include, among others, cardiac issues, depression, stroke, and heart attacks.

Numerous studies have shown that when individuals get enough sleep, they feel better and perform better. According to sleep specialists, also raise the likelihood that they will live longer, healthier, and more successful lives.

Avoiding alcohol, caffeine, and nicotine can help you beat insomnia. Naturally, all of these will eventually make the mind restless. Caffeine will make the mind seem to be more active than it is.

Most individuals choose stimulants because they need the energy to start their day. Caffeine is one of the stimulants nowadays to guarantee alertness and wakefulness in the morning and throughout the day. However, they lack knowledge that coffee is one of the main contributors to sleeplessness. The equilibrium between awake and sleep is disrupted.

Therefore, insomniacs should avoid these beverages for a good night's sleep. You could struggle to fall and stay asleep at night if you don't take that coffee break and instead go for a glass of plain water.

In addition, one of the finest self-help methods for insomnia is creating a sleep regimen for yourself. It is a crucial step towards permanently conquering insomnia.

The body requires consistency, so go to bed at the same time each night and get up at the same time each morning. The human body enjoys routine. It benefits from habit. Your body is more likely to remain on track with regular sleep and wake-up times. Avoid rotating schedules, late-night events, night shifts, and other activities that can interfere with your sleep routine.

Try drinking a glass of warm milk if you have trouble falling asleep. There is evidence that this conventional insomnia treatment may improve your sleep quality. Milk includes an amino acid called tryptophan, which helps prevent hunger from interrupting sleep.

Serotonin, a "relaxing" molecule, is produced in the brain from dopamine. Calcium has a strong pro-metabolic effect, lowering stress and parathyroid hormone levels and contributing to sleeplessness.

Not only that, but you can always change your daily routine to allow time for meditation or yoga. Numerous studies have shown that yoga and meditation may significantly enhance sleep patterns. It's crucial to take time for oneself to unwind. You may practice these methods in the privacy and comfort of your own home. It facilitates increased overall body flexibility, mental relaxation, and physical de-stressing. Aim to practice yoga or meditation for at least 30 minutes each day. Yoga and meditation are often best practiced in the early morning, in a serene setting, and while exposed to sunshine.

All you need to do to meditate is to sit still and quiet your thoughts. To help you relax, try listening to soothing music. The mind will be able to unwind more quickly at night, and you will have an easier time falling asleep if you become acclimated to meditation during the day.

As for yoga, you may either practice at home for more privacy or attend yoga sessions with plenty of people. It will improve your sleep in a variety of ways. The practice of certain yoga poses will improve blood flow to the brain's sleep region, which has the impact of restoring a regular sleep cycle.

Remember that sleep is a natural and essential function, not a luxury or way of life. Find the fundamental reasons, alter your diet, sip some warm milk, establish a sleeping regimen, do yoga, and meditate. If you follow the abovementioned suggestions, you'll finally obtain the rest you need.

Chapter 6

Turning It Off

Battling Insomnia

The struggle against sleeplessness is difficult. When treating insomnia, you attempt to prevent your thoughts from being too busy at night. There is no cause to be terrified of wondering whether everything will end for endless nights in a row.

The only thing worrying will do is keep you up at night. So give up fighting your mental insomnia! All you have to do is tell your monkey brain to shut down.

You want your thoughts to become more relaxed at night so you can sleep easily. A good night's rest and being fully aware the following day are made possible by getting the recommended quantity of sleep. People may have trouble falling asleep because their monkey brains won't shut down.

Instead, they begin obsessing about pointless ideas that prevent them from going to sleep. Turning off requires practice. Many busy folks only think about their life before going to sleep! Now and again, it's beneficial to reflect, but not just before bed. This is often the main thing preventing you from falling asleep.

Therefore, if you want to reflect on your life, try getting up earlier so you have time in the morning or set aside some time in the evening.

Stressful night = Poor Sleep

Another reason individuals struggle to fall asleep is that they engage in too many overstimulating activities at night, which keeps them up instead of making them feel weary. Some people even like drinking coffee at night! Why are individuals having trouble sleeping? Therefore, avoid using your laptop, mobile device, or television before bed. Avoid engaging in mentally and physically demanding activities late at night. Avoid the

'Blue-screen' on your electrical gadgets, which is essential.

Never again skip a night of sleep.

Setting a sleep routine is a further effective sleep strategy. Most individuals avoid doing it. They choose to just go to sleep when they are exhausted instead. Instead, kids should establish a pattern and set a time for going to bed. Your mind will eventually get trained to shut down when bedtime comes around.

A consistent sleep schedule is the greatest way to guarantee greater sleep quality. In actuality, consistency and a regular sleep pattern are beneficial to our health. Although there isn't a single effective remedy, maintaining a regular sleep schedule will undoubtedly aid in permanently overcoming chronic insomnia.

Switching off at Night: How To Do It

Turning off electronic gadgets should be your first step after supper and before you finish cleaning up for the evening. When you are getting ready for bed, having your phone or computer on will excite your brain, ultimately preventing you from falling asleep. Recognize that using your technological gadgets is addicting and that you won't be able to quit.

The light will disrupt your sleep cycle and keep you up all night. It is advised to put all electronic devices away at least one hour before night.

It's okay to read before bed, but not on your electronics. Before night, reading a physical book as a pastime might aid in preparing you for sleep. It's best to avoid reading in bed. You're advised not to read in the room where you need to go to sleep since you don't want your thoughts to be active there. Once again, program your mind to shut down when you enter your bedroom. It's okay to read a book while lying in bed if you can relax totally while doing so. If not, it's preferable to read somewhere else.

The next thing you may do is put on some music and make a note of any reminders you'll need for the next day. You can reduce your tension and quiet your thoughts with music. Try to choose music with a mellower, slower beat. Anything noisy or thrilling excites your thoughts, making it more difficult for you to sleep. For instance, listening to classical music will put you in a far calmer mood than listening to rock music.

Another suggestion is to schedule your days before going to bed. It helps cleanse your thoughts and write down to-do lists for the next day.

Your mind will remain busy if you remain awake in bed while repeatedly telling yourself that you must recall something. Consider your notebook as a "dump it and forget it" vault. Just take some paper and write down a few notes. You'll be able to relax and sleep more easily as a result.

Another thing you may do is to have a calming beverage, like tea, just before going to bed. However, be careful to avoid coffee, alcohol, and beverages with a lot of sugar. Your body and mind may both relax with a lovely cup of tea.

This is also a great approach to giving yourself time. A moment to unwind and calm down. This may be carried out while reading or listening to music. If tea isn't your thing, consider having a snack before bed. Avoid foods that are hard to digest and too heavy in calories. Whatever the case, taking a little snack before bed is a good idea since occasionally hunger is the only cause of difficulty falling asleep.

Lowering the temperature in your room is another approach to guarantee sound sleep. Setting your bedroom's thermostat a little lower is the most effective approach to do this. Our bodies are programmed to indicate when it is time to rest when we enter a colder environment.

Why not also take a brief shower just before going to bed? To quickly chill down, choose a cold shower. If not, consider investing in a bed fan, a cooler mattress, or a little stroll before bed.

You may include all of the activities above in your nightly ritual. Try them out and see which suits you and your schedule the best. You won't have any problem falling asleep or staying asleep again in no time.

Conclusion

With any luck, this book can help you quit or avoid sleeplessness. You are welcome to use any advice and methods this book suggests to guarantee a sound night's sleep. After all, a good night's sleep is essential for your physical and emotional health. All of them, whether they are man-made or natural remedies, lifestyle adjustments, or routine-setting, help to avoid insomnia.

What should we do next? It's time to act right now!

Whichever approach you find to be most effective for you, add it to your regular regimen. Imagine your typical day after incorporating these tactics into your routine as you write them down.
You can only determine which method works best to combat insomnia by trying them out.

About The Author

Jennifer Schwarz is the owner and creator of Kenvi Consulting, which offers a wide variety of services to help you be as successful as possible. She's passionate about helping people get healthy and happy. Jennifer loves yoga, music, and teaching people how to be their best selves. She's also the writer behind Pure Yoga: Mastering the healing art for Health and Peacefulness, Organize your life: A most efficient method to organize your life, The untapped gold mine of Diet, weight loss, and many more.

She is not a nutritionist or trained chef, just a determined mom who searched high and low for a way of eating that would reduce inflammation and live a happy and healthy life.

Jennifer lives in Dallas, Texas, with her husband and two beautiful children.

Other Books By Jennifer Schwarz

1. 350 Low Carb Cookbook: Quick and Delicious Low Carb Recipes Can Help You Lose Weight Effortlessly
2. DIETING AND WEIGHT LOSS: 5 Unexpected Dieting and Weight Loss Tips
3. Pure Yoga: Mastering The Healing Art For Health And Peacefulness
4. TOP KETOGENIC DIET: The Quickest & Easiest Way To weight loss
5. 14 Days: To A Better KETOGENIC, DIET
6. Organize Your Life: Most Efficient Method To Organize Your Life
7. A Guide To KETO, DIETING At Any Age: A Perfect Guide to Losing Weight, Boost Your Energy and Eating Healthy
8. Super Health For Super Kids: Parenting Guides For Picky Eating And Stronger Immune System
9. Respect All Life: Tasty Vegetarian Food And Cooking
10. Healthy Juicing: Exploring the Science, Nutrition, and Impact of Juicing on Your Health and Well-being
11. Natural Herbal Medicine: Exploring The Benefits, Safety, and Effectiveness of Herbal Medications
12. Herbal Tea Remedies: Transform Your Health With The Magic Of Herbal Tea

One Last Thing…

Dear Reader,

I hope you enjoyed reading this book and found it to be valuable for your needs. As an author, it means a lot to me when readers take the time to leave a review on Amazon. Your feedback not only helps me improve my writing but also helps potential readers decide if this book is right for them.

If you have a few minutes to spare, I would greatly appreciate it if you could leave a review on Amazon. Your honest opinion can help other readers make informed decisions and can make a real difference in the success of this book.

To leave a review, simply search for the book title and my name on Amazon.com, and select the book from the search results. Once you have navigated to the book's page, scroll down to the review section and share your thoughts on the book.

Rest assured that every single review is personally read and appreciated by me. Your feedback is crucial in helping me understand what worked well and what could be improved upon in future editions. Thank you in advance for your support and for taking the time to leave a review.

Best regards,

Jennifer Schwarz